HERBS FOR CLEARING THE SKIN

When an eruption appears on the skin it is a sign that something is wrong internally. This book gives blood purifying herbal remedies for dealing with boils, eczema, pimples, shingles, warts, and many other skin complaints.

HERBS FOR CLEARING THE SKIN

by
SARAH BECKETT

Drawings by Jill Fry

THORSONS PUBLISHERS LIMITED
Wellingborough, Northamptonshire

First published 1973
Seventh Impression 1984

ISBN 0 7225 0211 7

Printed and bound in Great Britain by
Richard Clay (The Chaucer Press) Ltd.,
Bungay, Suffolk.

CONTENTS

THE FUNCTIONS AND DISEASES OF THE SKIN

When all is well, and the body has a pure bloodstream, plus good wholesome food, any eruptions of the skin are very unlikely.

The skin has many jobs to perform, and only if it is healthy can they be done with maximum benefit.

The skin must be able to absorb from the air and sunshine just as efficiently as it exudes perspiration and poisons. It should also be smooth and elastic.

If the body has efficient circulation and the blood is pure, this is reflected in healthy pink cheeks and a smooth skin, without blemishes.

On the other hand, if there are things wrong internally, then the skin is one of the first visible signs, because when the normal channels for expelling waste material are not working efficiently, that is, the kidneys or bowels, they become inadequate and then the skin is called upon to undertake an elimination. Many people are constipated and this can cause all kinds of skin blemishes.

An eruption takes place at the easiest point of exit, according to the type of toxic material that has to be eliminated.

People who are always taking drugs have many skin troubles; the body is constantly trying to rid the system of their poisons. Then there are those who eat vast amounts of white sugar which creates much acid in the system, and again the body tries to throw out the poisons through the skin. And the people suffering from nerves and nervous tension do not escape; this group also have skin troubles and so do those who rarely perspire, who never take sufficient exercise and wear so many clothes that the skin cannot work properly.

When an eruption of any kind breaks out on the skin it is a sign and should be a warning that something is wrong internally.

To treat the skin itself is putting the cart before the horse, but if the basic cause is dealt with, and the bloodstream is cleaned up, then the symptoms on the skin, whatever they may be called will disappear.

If a carbuncle or boil develops an improvised channel has been made for the outlet of decomposed cells, pus, acids and other debris, which normally would be excreted through the urine and the bowel, as a gas via the lungs and internal flatus.

Nature is a wonderful balancer, and if we think for one moment, *everything* in nature is balanced. So if anything goes wrong healthwise she tries very hard to adjust and often this means that the poisons are disgorged through the skin.

One of the reasons why there is an increase in skin eruptions is because of all the medical injections and antibiotics, steroids, serums and vaccines plus all the pills and capsules taken by mouth.

Some cosmetics too can be dangerous to the skin because they contain mercurial salts, arsenic, copper and sulphates. But there are some preparations on the market to-day made from natural ingredients, such as herbs and oils which are more wholesome.

Many names are given to skin eruptions: dermatitis is one that is very commonly used and it simply means inflammation of the skin and loosely covers a number of skin troubles.

Acne is very prevalent among young people at present, mainly because they live on too much sugar and a refined diet.

Blood must be well cleansed and diet watched. These topics are discussed later in this book. However, if acne is ignored, in two or three years this eruption can become very severe and a break-up of the under layers of the skin takes place. Holes and pockmarks appear and remain long after the last spot of acne has gone, sometimes for many years. Usually acne appears only on the face, chest and upper back.

Boils are very painful swellings, which are dark red or mauvish. The matter forms into a single core and when ready, this comes away and the pus drains out.

A carbuncle is similar in appearance to a boil but does not protrude above the surface of the skin to quite the same extent, and it is deeper. A carbuncle oozes its pus from several channels, and not one, like a boil.

Eczema should be diagnosed by a qualified practitioner; it has several different medical names according to its appearance and locality. In recent years we have other types of eczema from cortizone, penicillin, and other drugs.

With any of these conditions, however, it is essential if possible to ascertain what triggered off the outbreak, because where there is an effect there must be a cause. It could come from food toxins, deficiencies, excess acidity or taking into the body harmful medicaments.

Itching is a predominent symptom and may be severe. Eczema reacts badly to sunshine, sea air and salt water. However, psoriasis is another very common skin complaint and it should be properly diagnosed because it looks very much like one form of eczema but sunshine, sea air and salt water do not make this condition any worse. It seems to be most prevalent in the autumn and winter. In most cases itching is almost incessant and it is often worse at night.

Shingles is a deep seated skin complaint called Herpes Zoster and it always follows the line of the nerve or nerves affected. Blisters erupt and then fill with pus and blood when scabs form. It is exceedingly painful and often lasts a long time.

Urticaria is a form of skin eruption which develops inflammatory wheals. This trouble can be acute or chronic; it is very distressing because the irritation is so severe. The wheals can come up quickly on any part of the body and last for a few minutes or an hour (it does not often go on much longer) and then they will disappear just as quickly. More wheals however, form on another part of the body on the same or next day, depending upon the severity of the attack.

Warts can appear anywhere on the body and they can be flat, large, small, seed-like, or horny. Again, a wart is an indication that all is not right internally. They should never be tampered with by cauterization or cutting.

In giving constitutional treatment many skin troubles clear up and many warts disappear.

2

HOW HERBS CAN CLEAR THE SKIN

Once again we look to herbs for the safe treatment of all skin troubles.

It is particularly important to remember what has been said in section 1; that is, symptoms on the skin come from some internal cause; they are an indication that something is wrong within.

Nothing is spontaneous. In other words, everything must have a beginning and an end, and every disease must have a cause and an effect.

When all is not well within the body, nature does her best to eliminate poisons and as the skin is the largest eliminative organ eruptions appear in various forms. Thus, it is not difficult to understand that if this form of elimination is cut short, it is to the detriment of the sufferer.

To treat spots, pimples, carbuncles, boils and other eruptions and sores, is only to touch the effect, leaving the cause intact. But this is not all. If ointments and salves made from cortizone or antibiotics are used freely, they clear the surface of the trouble but push back the poisons into the system, thus courting more troubles for the future. If treatment is given with herbal medicines, however, a different result will be achieved.

Herbs usually exert influences .in more than one direction and it will be noticed that, as well as being useful in skin troubles, nearly all the herbs discussed in this book also purify the blood, and so in this way it may be that all or part of the cause is removed.

In addition, herbs contain mineral salts, vitamins and foods for the body, all in their natural form. These are so vital to the human system that after taking herbs for a time, most patients begin to have a sense of well-being.

It may be asked at this point, 'Why, in the pages of this book, recommend applying certain herbs to the skin as poultices, fomentations or washes?' The answer is that herbs do not suppress if applied to the skin, but they can soothe and remove inflammations, or promote suppuration when necessary, and help the healing processes.

Curative processes take place from within the body when the patient is treated with herbs. They assist the system to eliminate all the poisons that are causing the trouble. Sometimes a reaction takes place in the form of diarrhoea or sneezing and running from the nose, but these symptoms do not last very long and the patient feels better afterwards, because the body is gradually being cleansed.

It is therefore wise to remember that if anything appears on the skin as a rash, an eruption, boil or carbuncle, the thing not to do is to clear the skin by suppressing these symptoms, because more trouble is sure to return at some later date; instead, use simple herbal medicines that have been used since man was put on earth,. as they are safe, gentle in action and curative.

BILBERRY
(*Vaccinium myrtillus*)

Also known as Whortleberry, Whinberry, Blaeberry, Truckleberry and Blackhearts.

Description: The berries grow on a small, branched shrub which has small, rose red wax-like flowers, followed by dark blue berries.

Part used: The berries.

Bilberry juice will stain linen or paper purple.

The berries are delicious in a fruit pie eaten with cream.

Bilberry extract is very useful as an application for

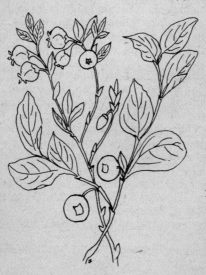

treating skin diseases such as scaly eczema and other
eczemas which are not moist or pustulous. It is also good
for burns and scalds.

Directions for use: Some extract should be spread
thickly on the cleansed skin with a soft sterile brush, and
covered with a thin layer of cotton wool and held with a
bandage. Change the dressing daily.

BITTERSWEET
(Solanum dulcamara)

Also known as Woody nightshade, Wolfe grape, Violet
broom, Scarlet berry, Nightshade vine, Fever twig,
Felonwood, Staff Vine.

Description: Grows commonly in moist and shady
places. This plant readily climbs up a support. It has
woody stalks with many creeping branches by which it
climbs up through hedges. It has long pointed leaves.
The flowers are small and grow in clusters, which are
purple with rather large yellow anthers. Bittersweet has
oval scarlet berries. The greenish-brown shoots are
indistinctly angular about ½ inch thick, sometimes
warty.

Part used: Year old greenish-brown shoots.

The name 'bittersweet' is due to the fact that if
chewed the stem at first tastes bitter, then sweet.

Culpeper says, 'It is good to remove Witchcraft both
in men and beast, as all sudden diseases whatsoever'.

This herb is excellent for all skin troubles; at the same
time it will purify the blood.

It makes the skin and kidneys active, thus eliminating
poisons.

Burns and scalds respond well when bathed with this
herb.

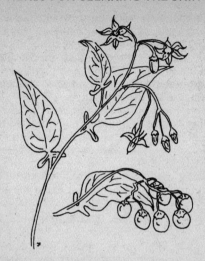

Directions for use: The fluid extract should be purchased and 1 teaspoonful taken in a little water at night and in the morning.

BROOKLIME
(Veronica beccabunga)

Also known as Water pimpernel.
Description: It grows commonly in brooks and ditches as a succulent plant. It has a creeping root which sends up stems at every joint. The smooth leaves are in pairs, rather broad and round. Its short stems grow from the main one with many small blue flowers that consist of five small round pointed petals.
Part used: The herb.

'It is eaten', says Gerard, 'in sallads as watercresses are.'

Culpeper says, 'It serves to purge the blood and body from all ill humours that would destroy health, and is helpful in scurvy'.

Amongst other things, this plant contains tannin, a pungent volatile oil, and sulphur.

The leaves, well washed and bruised, form a poultice for applying externally to ulcers, burns and whitlows.

Frequent doses of the infusion of this herb are helpful for those suffering from boils, abscesses and pimples.

Directions for use: An infusion of the leaves is made by adding 1 pint of boiling water to 1 oz. of the dried herb and when cold, a wineglassful should be taken frequently.

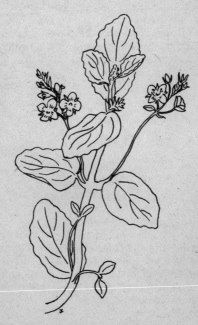

BUCKBEAN
(Menyanthes trifolata)

Also known as Bog-bean, Marsh trefoil, Water shamrock.
Description: It grows on marsh ground and on the
margins of woodlands. The leaves grow alternately on
stalks. The leaflets are three equal inversely egg-shaped
and wavelike. The flower stalk supports a stalked cluster
of pink flowers, fringed within the corolla. It creeps in
every direction as it has long rooting stems.
Part used: The herb.

An old Botanist said this herb was equal in beauty to
the kalmias, rhododendrons and exotic heaths on which

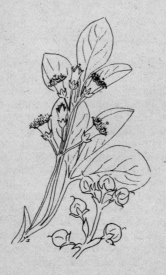

so much money is expended, whilst buckbean is disregarded.

'The root of the buckbean, or more properly it's creeping rhizomes, contain a large amount of farinaceous matter resembling starch. In Lapland and Finland these rhizomes are washed to free them from the bitter principle, powdered and made into bread. It is described as not being very palatable but possessed of considerable nutritive qualities.' From *Useful Plants of Great Britain*.

This herb is a somewhat bitter tonic which is excellent for skin diseases, especially for those that have a rheumatic foundation.

Directions for use: An infusion is made by pouring 1 pint of boiling water on to 1 oz. of the herb; this should be strained when cold and a wineglassful taken frequently.

BURDOCK
(Arctium lappa)

Also known as Lappa Hill, Beggars Burr, Thorny Burr, Clotbur, Hardock, Larebur, Turkey Burr, Personata and Happy Major. The burs of this dock are sometimes called Cockle buttons, Cuckle buttons, Beggar's buttons.

Description: This plant grows in large quantities in fairly damp places, along roadsides and about old buildings on waste ground. The root is brownish-grey and has a slightly sweet taste. The stem grows from 3 to 4 feet; the leaves are large, often 18-20 inches long, and look rather like those of rhubarb and they are whitish underneath. The flowers are like thistles and purple in colour and grow on short stems often at the leaf joint. They are globular with burs that can stick to clothing. The fruits (erroniously called seeds) are brownish-grey and wrinkled. The leaves and stems have a bitter taste.

Part used: The herb, root and seeds (fruits).

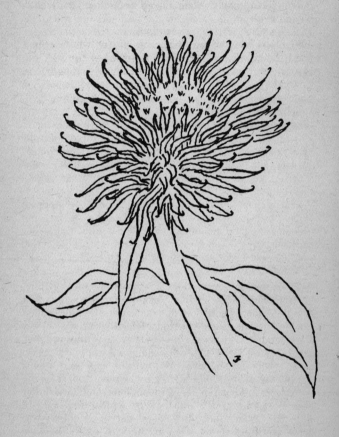

The botanical name Arctium is derived from *arklos*, a bear relating to the roughness of the burs, and Lappa is from *labein*, to seize.

The young stalks were boiled and eaten in salads in olden days.

Culpeper said: 'The Burdock leaves are cooling, moderately drying and discussing withal, whereby it is good for old ulcers and sores . . . the leaves bruised with the white of an egg and applied to any place burnt with fire, taketh out the fire, gives sudden ease, and heals it up afterwards'.

This herb is one of the best blood purifiers, it rapidly cleanses and eliminates impurities from the blood.

The seeds of this plant are very efficacious and have a great influence on the skin as they are of a very oily nature. They affect both the sebacious and the sudo-riferous glands, and they restore smoothness and a healthy action to the skin.

Burdock tea will, if taken freely, clear all kinds of skin troubles such as boils, carbuncles, burns and wounds. A very old herbalist said he found it almost a specific remedy for psoriasis, if drop doses of the fluid extract were taken regularly for 2 to 3 months.

Burdock has affected a cure in many cases of eczema and it is on record that after nearly two years of suffering a patient, who had tried nearly everything else, had her skin cleared in four weeks after taking this herb.

The root in decoction is an excellent remedy for skin troubles of the scaly, itching, vesicular, pimply and ulcerative character.

By cleansing the blood styes on the eyelids, boils and carbuncles are prevented.

Directions for use: Both root and seed may be taken as a decoction of 1 oz. to 1½ pints of water boiled down to a pint. A wineglassful should be taken 3 or 4 times daily. 10 to 20 drops of the fluid extract seed should be taken in water three times daily. A tea is made by infusing ½ oz. of the herb in ¼ pint of boiling water for fifteen minutes. A wineglass of the fluid should be taken after every meal.

CELANDINE
(Chelidonium majus)

Also known as Garden celandine, Greater celandine, Swallow-wort, Tetter-wort.

Description: It is very common and grows on old walls, amongst ruins and on waste ground. It is one of the herbs that has followed man and is more often found near his dwelling than in secluded places. It grows about 2 ft high, is slightly hairy, and the stems are brittle and full of a bright yellow juice. The leaves are feathery, greyish underneath, from 6 to 12 inches long and 2 to 3 inches wide. Leaflets grow opposite, deeply cut with

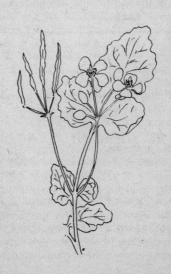

rounded teeth. The flowers are bright yellow with four petals in a calyx of two hollow parts. Black shining seeds are contained in narrow pods.

Part used: The herb.

The name chelidonium comes from the Greek word *Chelidon* — meaning a swallow — because of an ancient tradition that the bird makes use of this herb to open the eyes of it's young, or restore their sight if lost.

'If the yellow juice of the stalk of the celandine is applied to warts or corns after they have been gently scraped, it will cure them promptly and painlessly', says Dr. Fernie.

This herb is an excellent liver remedy and in turn will help skin troubles to clear up. It has been used in cases of eczema when there has been liver trouble as well.

Directions for use: 1 pint of boiling water should be poured on to 1 oz. of the dried herb and strained when cold. A wineglassful should be taken three times daily.

The fresh herb should be gathered and the stem cut, when the yellow juice will be released and can be used for corns and warts.

CHICKWEED
(Stellaria media)

Also known as Starweed, Stitchwort, Adder's mouth.

Description: This herb grows in hedges and ditches, in waste places, by the roadside, and in gardens. The stems are jointed with a line of fine hairs down one side only. The leaves grow opposite, are oval about ½ inch long and ¼ inch broad, the lower ones on stalks, the upper springing from the stem, they spread upwards and escape being overshadowed by other broad-leaved plants. The flowers grow singly in the axils of the upper leaves, the petals are white with a silvery-grey tint and they look like stars.

Part used: The herb.

It is called *Stellaria media*, a floral star of middle magnitude.

This herb grows all over the world and serves as food for small birds such as finches and linnets. Gerard translates an old herbal 'Little birds in cages are refreshed with chickweed when they loath their meat'.

Lord Bacon who watched carefully all the changes in nature said of this herb: 'When the flower expands boldly and fully, no rain will happen for four hours or upwards; if it continues in that open state, no rain will disturb the summer's day; but if it entirely shuts up or veils the white flower with its green mantle, let the traveller put on his great-coat, and the ploughman, with his beast of draught, expect rest from their labour'.

Culpeper said: 'It is a fine, soft, pleasing herb . . . The herb bruised or the juice applied with cloths or sponges dipped therein is effectual for all redness in the face, wheals, pushes, itch, scabs . . . '

Fernie said: 'This small herb abounds in the earthy salts of potash, which are admirable against scurvy when thus found in nature's laboratory, and a continued deprivation from which always proves disastrous to mankind'.

An infusion of this herb purifies the blood, and this is helpful in curing all skin diseases.

Chickweed soothes and heals anything in which it comes in contact: therefore, an ointment made from this herb is used freely on all kinds of wounds, inflamed skin, boils, burns and scalds.

For any skin sores, a chickweed herb bath will help, followed by an application of the ointment.

Directions for use: A tea is made by steeping a heaped teaspoonful of the dried herb for half-an-hour in a cup of boiling water. A cupful should be sipped slowly three or four times daily plus one at bedtime.

For external use a handful of the herb should be

boiled in 2 quarts of water for ten minutes and this should then be used as a body wash.

Chickweed ointment is obtainable from most Health Food Stores.

For a bath, about 1 lb of the herb should be chopped up and from 6 to 8 pints of boiling water poured on to it. It should be steeped for thirty minutes and then added to warm (not hot) bath water. This can be repeated every other day.

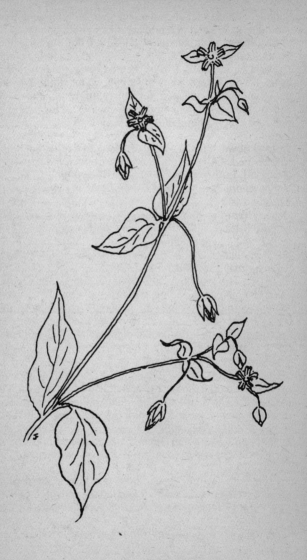

CLIVERS
(Galium aparine)

Also known as Cleavers, Goose-grass, Mutton-chops, Catchweed, Clitheren, Goose-bill, Robin-run-in-the-grass, Burweed, Loveman, Clithers, Goose-heriff, and Clite.

Description: This herb grows freely in fields, on waste land and is a 'scrambler over hedges'. This is one of the square-stemmed herbs. It grows from the whorl of sharp serrated leaves like the rough-edged mandibles of a goose.

These leaves are in whorls of six about ½ inch long and ¼ inch broad with backward, bristly hairs at the margins. The fruit is nearly globular, about $\frac{1}{8}$th inch in diameter, which with the stems are covered with little hooks so that they can catch into the wool of sheep and so get dispersed. They also attach themselves to people's clothing. The plant fastens itself in a ladder-like manner to shrubs growing around so that it can get up through the hedgerows and into light.

Part used: The herb.

This herb is also called Harriff or Erriff from the Anglo-Saxon 'hedge-rife', a tax gatherer or robber because it plucks wool from the sheep as they pass through the hedge.

The botanical name *Aparine* has the same meaning as Grip-grass being derived from the Greek verb *apairo*, to lay hold of.

The term Galium comes from the Greek word *gala*, milk, and the plant family of Bedstraws, of which Clivers is one, were formerly employed to 'curdle' milk instead of rennet.

A red dye can be made from the root of this herb.

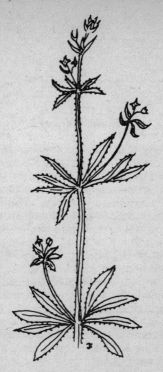

On analysis it is found that Clivers contains 3 distinct acids; tannic acid (of galls), citric acid (of lemons) and the special rubichloric acid of the plant.

It is an excellent blood purifier, especially if the leaves are eaten like spinach.

It is an excellent remedy for eczema and psoriasis and it makes a good face wash to clear the complexion.

It can stop the bleeding of wounds.

Directions for use: An infusion can be made by pouring 1 pint of hot or cold water on to 1 oz. of the herb and after standing for fifteen minutes a wineglassful should be taken frequently.

DANDELION
(Taraxacum officinalis)

Also known as Blowball, Timetable, Wiggers, Swinesnout.

Description: This herb grows everywhere in pastures, meadows, on waste ground, and is well known as a weed in our gardens. The stems grow to a height of about 6 inches and there is one flower to each stem. The leaves have jagged edges which resemble the jaw of a lion fully supplied with teeth. The root is long, dark brown and very bitter, but not disagreeably so.

Part used: Leaves and root.

Some old writers say that this herb has been named from the heraldic lion which is vividly yellow with teeth of gold. In short, a dandy lion.

The herb has been known to the Arabian physicians since the eleventh century when it was called taraxacon. This name is the Arabian corruption of the Greek *trogimon*, meaning edible, or it may have been derived from the Greek *taraxos* meaning 'disorder' and *akos*, remedy.

Fernie said: 'It once happened that a plague of insects destroyed the harvest in the island of Minorca so that the inhabitants had to eat the wild produce of the country, and many of them subsisted for some while entirely on this plant'.

The root of dandelion makes a good substitute for coffee when roasted and ground. It may be purchased in tins and is delicious made as ordinary coffee and it has many health giving properties.

The dandelion contains twenty-eight parts of Sodium and it is a very good blood purifier. At the same time, it will destroy acid in the blood and thus bring about a better balance where necessary; many patients have too much acid in their bloodstreams.

This herb is very good for all skin troubles, especially for eczema.

There is a prescription for all skin troubles which includes agrimony, gentian or buckbean, sea holly and ginger as well as dandelion.

Directions for use: Boil 2 ozs. of the root or herb in 1 quart of water down to 1 pint, a wineglassful should be taken every three hours.

To make the prescription mentioned above take:

        ½ oz. Dandelion root
        ½ oz. Agrimony
        ½ oz. Sea Holly
        ½ oz. English Gentian or Buckbean
        ¼ oz. lump Ginger, crushed

add to 3 pints of water and boil down to 1½ pints, strain and when cold a wineglassful should be taken three or four times daily.

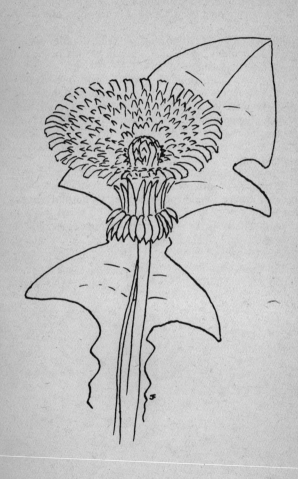

ECHINACEA
(Echinacea angustifolia)

Also known as Purple cone flower, Sampson root, Kansas niggerhead, Black sampson.

Description: Root greyish-brown, twisted. This is imported; it is native to the prairie regions of America, west of Ohio.

Part used: The root.

Echinacea must be included in this small work because of its wonderful properties to clear and purify the blood.

It is excellent in all skin eruptions, especially for

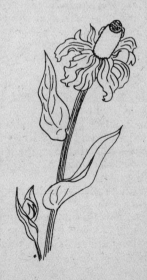

carbuncles, boils, bites and stings of poisonous insects, sores and wounds.
Directions for use: The fluid extract should be purchased and 30 drops taken in water three times daily.

FUMITORY
(Fumaria officinalis)

Also known as Earth smoke, Horned poppy, Wax dolls.
Description: This herb grows freely in waste places and often in cornfields. It is a slender, straggling plant with divided leaves of a bluish-green colour. Many pink flowers in short spikes grow on a common erect stalk.
Part used: The herb.

Fumitory is named from the Latin *fumus*, earth smoke, which refers either to the appearance of it's lovely foliage or to the belief that it was produced, not from seed, but from vapours rising out of the earth. Pliny said: 'Just as smoke causes the eyes to water so also does fumitory, when applied to them, and hence its name'.

The name 'Wax dolls' is because of the rose-coloured flowers with the little dark purple heads which look very like the wax dolls of old.

Culpeper said: 'The juice of Fumitory and docks mingled with vinegar, and the places gently washed or wet therewith, cures all sorts of scabs, pimples, blotches, wheals and pushes which rise on the face or hands or any other part of the body'.

Gerard said: 'It helpeth in the summer time those that are troubled with scabs'.

This herb contains fumaric acid which is so useful in chronic skin eruptions with scabs, and pimples on the face and also for freckles. It helps to clear the skin of many troubles.

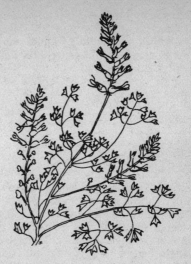

Directions for use: 1 pint of boiling water should be poured on to 1 oz. of the herb and when cold and strained a wineglassful should be taken three times daily, and more often in bad cases.

GARLIC
(Allium sativa)

Also known as Poor man's treacle, Churl's treacle and by the Greeks, *Skorodon.*
Description: This herb is found in many gardens and it looks rather like an onion. The bulb consists of several combined cloves and has an odour much stronger than onions.

Part used: The bulb.

This was first cultivated in English gardens in 1540. Garlic has been used as a medicine for thousands of years; the Babylonians, the Greeks and the Egyptians all held it in very high esteem. The worth attached to the garlic and the onion tribe by ancient Egyptians often elicited the sarcasm of the writers of other nations.

Fuller, referring to Garlic said: 'Not to speak of the murmuring Israelites, who prized it even before manna itself, some avow it soveraigne for men and beasts in most maladies, though the scent thereof be somewhat valiant and offensive. Indeed a large book is written on its virtues, which if held proportionate with truth, one would wonder any man should die, who hath garlic growing in his garden'.

Modern research has confirmed all claims made by the ancient peoples but, for our purpose, suffice it to say that garlic is a first class blood purifier, and in so doing, it will clear the skin of blotches, blemishes, pimples and it will help to rid the system of boils or carbuncles.

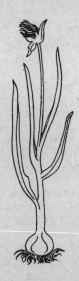

Culpeper said: 'Garlic takes away spots and blemishes in the skin'.

As it is such a cleansing remedy, garlic should be taken by all those who suffer from any skin conditions, as it will supplement and help any other medicines.

Many people are reluctant to eat garlic because of it's strong odour, which persists for a considerable time. However, it is now possible to obtain capsules of garlic which, when swallowed, overcome to a large degree, the unpleasantness associated with the taking of this herb.

Directions for use: Capsules of garlic should be purchased and taken according to directions on the bottle.

HOUSELEEK
(Sempervivum tectorum)

Also known as Stonecrop, Sengreen, Jupiter's Eye, Thors Beard.

Description: This little herb grows plentifully on walls and tops of small buildings. The leaves form rosettes 2 to 3 inches in diameter; they are fleshy and flat with no stalk; oblong, incurved and pointed, hairy on the margins. It bears small purple flowers on long stems.

Part used: Fresh leaves. Houseleek is derived from the anglo-saxon word *leek*, a plant growing on a house.

This little plant has great tenacity and vitality and it is recorded that a botanist tried hard for eighteen months to dry a plant of houseleek for his herbarium but failed. He restored it to its first site where it grew again as though nothing had interfered with its ordinary life.

In olden times it was often planted on roofs of houses because it is supposed to be a guard against thunder and lightning.

The Greeks were very fond of houseleeks and grew them in vases in the windows of their houses.

Galen extolled the uses of houseleek in the treatment of erysipelas and shingles.

In rural districts the bruised leaves of the fresh plant were often applied to burns, scalds, sore legs and chronic skin diseases.

Gerard said: 'The juice being gently rubbed on any place stung by nettles or bees, or bitten by any venemous creature doth presently take away the pain'.

The juice is very helpful in curing corns and warts, if applied daily.

Parkinson said: 'The juice takes away corns from tne toes and feet if they be bathed therewith every day, and at night emplastered as it were, with the skin of the same houseleek'.

Directions for use: The fresh leaves are bruised and applied as a poultice to inflammatory conditions of the skin.

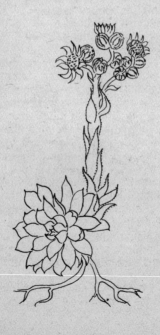

LADY'S MANTLE
(Alchemilla vulgaris)

Also known as Lion's Foot, Great sanicle.
Description: This herb grows in pastures and woodlands. The leaves are rounded and are about 2 inches in diameter and have nine obtuse serrate lobes on slender stalks of about 4 inches long. The whole plant is covered with soft downy hairs. The flowers are green on a forked stem which has small three-lobed leaves at the base of each fork. It grows to about 1 ft high.
Part used: The herb.

The Arabian physycians have a very high opinion of

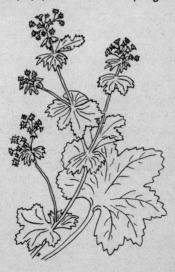

the remedial virtues of this common species and Hoffman and others have confirmed that it has the power of restoring beauty and freshness to the faded complexion.

Culpeper said: 'It is also a good wound-herb both inwardly and outwardly, by drinking a decoction or bathing and fomenting, for it dries up the humidity of sores and heals inflammation. It draws the corruption from, and heals green wounds; it cures all old sores'.

Lady's mantle should be used for all wounds, and for the after effects of accidents. It is excellent also for all blemishes of the skin.

Directions for use: An infusion should be made by pouring 1 pint of boiling water on to 1 oz. of the herb and a wineglassful taken three times daily. Any skin troubles may also be bathed with this liquid.

MARSHMALLOW
(Althaea officinalis)

Also known as Mallards, Schloss tea, Sweat weed, Althaea, Mortification root, Bull's eyes, Meshmellish, Soldier's buttons, Wild geranium.

Description: This common herb grows in damp places and near ditches, especially near the sea. The roots are many and long, shooting from one head the size of a thumb or finger. It has many soft, hairy, white stalks, 3 to 4 feet high, spreading with many branches; the leaves are soft and hairy, pointed and deeply serrated at the margins. The flowers are pink and grow in bunches.

Part used: The root and leaves.

Pliny said: 'Whosoever shall take a spoonful of the Mallows shall that day be free from all diseases that may come to him'.

The root is sweet and very mucilaginous when chewed, containing more than half its weight of saccharine viscous mucilage. This makes it very soothing, and able to subdue heat and irritation. If applied locally it helps the soreness of inflamed parts.

Marshmallow ointment is excellent, particularly for mollifying heat. In olden days men and women were given hot irons to hold to test their integrity. To do this they made an adhesive paste by mixing marshmallow juice with fleabane seed and the white of an hen's egg and when their hands were coated with it they could hold the glowing irons for a few minutes without any trouble.

Culpeper said: 'The juice of mallows boiled in old oil takes away roughness of the skin, scurf or dry scabs in the head or other parts if they be anointed with the decoction, and preserves the hair from falling. It is effective against scalds and burns, St. Anthony's fire and other hot and painful swellings in any part of the body. The leaves bruised or rubbed upon any place stung with bees, wasps or the like takes away pain, inflammation and swelling'.

This herb is excellent for all inflammations of the skin, and for sores and skin troubles generally. It cleanses and at the same time heals.

A poultice may be applied to the infected part made from the leaves or bathed with the infusion of either root or leaves.

Directions for use: An infusion or tea is made by adding a teacupful of boiling water to a teaspoonful of the leaves and infused for fifteen minutes then strained. A wineglassful may be taken 3 times daily.

A decoction of 1 oz. of root should be simmered in 1½ pints of water until 1 pint remains. A wineglassful should be taken 3 times daily.

Made up ointment is usually sold in Health Food Stores.

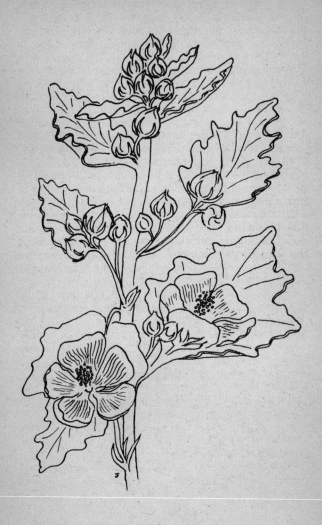

NETTLE
(Urtica dioica)

Also known as Stinging nettle, Common nettle.
Description: Grows on all waste ground. The stems are 2 to 3 feet high with opposite, stalked, oval leaves, serrated at the margins. The flowers are small, and green. It is recognised by its yellow, creeping root.
Part used: Flowers, leaves and seeds.

Urtica comes from *ob urendo* from burning as the leaves sting and burn when touched. The word nettle is derived from *net* which means something spun or sewn, and it indicates the thread made from the hairs of the

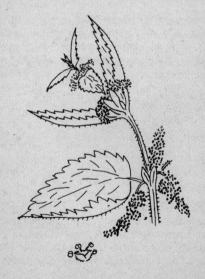

plant and formerly used by the people of the Scandinavian nations. Scottish weavers in the seventeenth century also used the nettle as 'Scotch cloth is only the housewifery of the nettle' said the historian Westmacott. The poet Campbell wrote: 'I have slept in nettle sheets, and dined off a nettle table cloth more durable than any other linen'.

Chlorophyll is generally obtained from nettles and many tons are gathered annually for that purpose.

The nettle contains iron, sulphur, potassium and sodium and it is therefore an excellent blood cleanser.

It is very good for eczema and nettle rash and all minor skin troubles. Nettle tea should be taken internally for these conditions.

If the tincture is applied to burns it will take the pain away immediately but it may have to be repeated.

In the spring if nettle tops are gathered and cooked as spinach they are not only delicious but will clean the blood of impurities. If the water in which nettles have been cooked is drunk, it will clear the skin of any blemishes.

Directions for use: Nettle tea should be made by adding 1 oz. of the herb or seed to 1 pint of boiling water. It should be left for at least five minutes and then taken as tea, or a wineglassful may be taken 3 times daily. It may be sweetened if desired.

PLANTAIN
(Plantago major)

Also known as Waybread, Soldiers, Hard-heads, Fighting-cocks. The Englishman's Foot and 'Whiteman's Foot as it has followed our colonists to all parts of the globe.

Description: This herb grows as a weed in fields and by

roadsides. Its broad, strongly veined leaves lie spread around its root-stock and from June to September its tall spikes of greenish flowers, or the brown ripened seeds which succeed them are conspicuous for all to see. The flower stalks are about a foot high.

Part used: The whole plant.

In the highlands this herb is called *slanus* a Gaelic word which means literally 'the plant of healing'. Plantago is probably derived from the Latin *planta*, the sole of the foot, because of the broad flat leaves lying close to the ground, and ago, the old word for wort, a cultivated plant.

Canaries love the spikes of seeds from this plant as do many wild birds. It is believed in some parts that toads cure themselves of their complaints by eating of the wayside plantain.

Culpeper says: 'One part of the herb water and two parts of the brine of powdered beef boiled together and clarified, is a remedy for all scabs and itching in the head and body, all manner of tetters, ringworm, the shingles and all manner of fretting sores. All the plantains are good wound herbs to heal fresh or old wounds or sores, either inward or outward'.

Dioscorides advised that the plantain should be applied externally to all kinds of sores.

Country people used to apply the leaves to open sores and wounds, and make poultices or hot fomentations to apply to the skin for any 'dirty' wounds, boils or carbuncles etc, and a hot decoction to drink.

This herb has a cooling, soothing effect in cases of sores and ulcers. It is very useful in erysipelas, eczema, burns and scalds.

Directions for use: The green leaves give wonderful relief if mashed up and applied as a poultice to any part of the body stung by poisonous insects, snake-bites, boils or carbuncles.

A tea for external use is made by pouring a pint of boiling water on to 1 oz. of the herb. It can be used as frequently as is necessary.

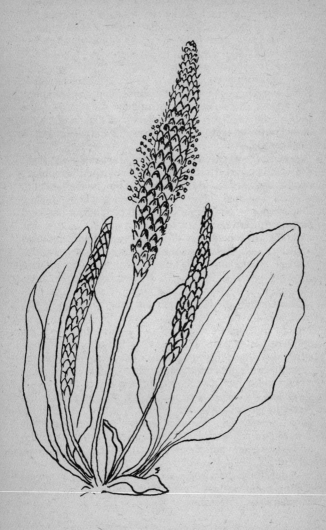

RED CLOVER
(Trifolium pratense)

Also known as Trefoil, Purple cloves, Suckles, Bee-bread, Cocksheads.

Description: It grows in grassland, fields and waysides. The flowers are purple-red in dense roundish oblong heads; the leaflets are broad, oval, or inversely heart--shaped, notched, often marked with a white crescent-shaped spot.

Part used: Flowers.

A field of clover may vie with a bean-field or the hop garden in sweetness of odour.

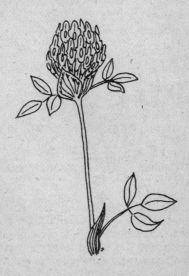

Clover is a corruption of the Latin *clava*, a club, and the 'clubs' on our playing cards are representations of clover leaves. It was introduced into England by Sir Richard Weston in 1645 and contains more nutriment for cattle than any other fodder.

This is a sensitive plant and Pliny said: 'Its leaves do start up as if afraid of an assault when tempestuous weather is at hand'.

Red clover contains, amongst other ingredients, silica and lime. It is an excellent blood purifier and helps the healing of fresh wounds and any sores. Skin eruptions of children respond well to this remedy: the affected parts should be bathed.

Directions for use: Use in place of tea and coffee and make as ordinary tea by adding 1½ pints of boiling water to 2 teaspoonsful of the dried flowers.

Any parts of the skin may be bathed with the tea.

SASSAFRAS
(Sassafras officinalis)

Also known as Ague tree, Saxifrax, Cinnamon wood.

Description: This is a native of Mexico and also grows from Canada to Florida. It is imported in the form of chips from the bark.

Part used: The bark of the root.

In the southern parts of America, where this tree grows abundantly, the scent perfumes the air for great distances around.

Sir Francis Drake first brought the roots of sassafras to this country from America and a tea made from it soon gained wide popularity as a cure for all ills. It was called 'saloop' and was served from many street stalls to English gentlemen who gathered in public to drink this

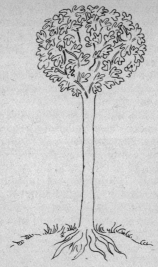

remarkable new health brew!

Sassafras is often called 'spring medicine' as it purifies the blood and cleanses the entire system. It is valuable in all skin diseases and eruptions.

Directions for use: 1 pint of boiling water should be poured on to 1 oz. of the crushed bark and infused for fifteen minutes. A wineglassful should be taken four or five times daily.

SCURVY GRASS
(Cochlearia officinalis)

Also known as Spoonwort.
Description: This herb grows on muddy seashores on an

angular smooth, shining stem 12 to 14 inches high with fleshy narrow green leaves and thick clusters of small white flowers which grow to about 10 inches in height. They have nearly globular seed pods. It has a salty taste. It is closely allied to watercress.

Part used: The herb.

The name spoonwort is given because the shape of the leaves resemble an old fashioned spoon.

'The scurvy grass was well known to early mariners as a remedy for scurvy which formerly proved so disastrous on long voyages. It was brought to notice by Captain Cook who used it in the Southern Seas.' — C. Pierpoint Johnson.

Culpeper said: 'Infused or the juice expressed, is better than the decoction, because the volatile parts are lost in boiling; it is a specific remedy against scurvy; it purifies the juices of the body from the bad effects of the distemper and clears the skin of scabs, pimples and foul eruptions'.

Scurvy grass contains potash salts. It is an excellent

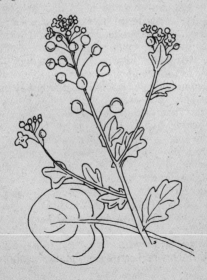

blood purifier and helpful in all skin eruptions, including sores, pimples, boils and abscesses.

The leaves are very wholesome in a spring salad.

Directions for use: An infusion is made by pouring 1 pint of boiling water on to 2 ozs. of the herb and when cold this should be strained. A wineglassful should be taken five or six times daily.

SHEPHERD'S PURSE
(Capsella bursa-pastoris)

Also known as Shepherd's Sprout, Mother's heart, Pick-pocket, Clapper's Pouch, Rattle Pouch.

Description: This is one of the most common wayside English weeds, but it grows also in most parts of the world. It has a rosette of leaves, deeply serrated on the ground level and a slender stem 10 to 15 inches tall, bearing a spike of small white flowers, followed by triangular flattened seed pods.

Part used: The whole plant.

Dr. Fernie said: 'This herb is of natural growth in most parts of the world, but varies in luxuriance according to soil and situation. Whilst thickly strewn over the whole surface of the earth, it faces alike the heat of the tropics and the rigours of the Arctic regions; even if trodden underfoot it rises again and again with ever-enduring vitality, as if designed to fulfil some special purpose in the far-seeing economy of nature'.

In some parts of England shepherd's purse is known as Clapper's pouch, referring to the licensed begging of lepers when in olden times they walked along with a bell and a clapper which was made of two or three boards which rattled, and so drew attention to passers by, not only that they were contageous but begging for alms

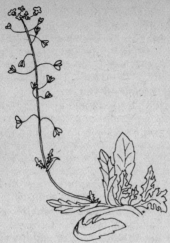

which was dropped into the pouches held out on long sticks.

Culpeper said, 'this herb is excellent for all wounds, especially wounds in the head'.

Shepherd's purse contains vitamin K. It is excellent for the skin and will stop all bleeding.

Directions for use: 1 pint of water should be poured on to 1 oz. of the dried herb and allowed to cool and then it should be strained. A wineglassful should be taken 3 times daily.

SOAPWORT
(Saponaria officinalis)

Also known as Soaproot, Bouncing Bet, Fuller's Herb, and formerly known as Bruisewort.

Description: Grows on roadsides and near woods in moist places. The leaves grow opposite, smooth and pointed, about two inches long and ¾ inch broad, greyish-green when dried. The flowers are pink and grow in clusters on stalks branching from the top of the main ones.

Part used: The leaves and root.

Gerard states: 'It is commonly called Saponaria, of the great scouring qualities of the leaves have; for they yield out of themselves a certaine juice when they are bruised, which scoureth almost as well as sope . . . .'

A soapy froth is obtained when a decoction is made of the root or leaves; this herb has been used by mendicant monks as a substitute for soap for washing their clothes as it will remove dirt and stains.

Soapwort is used extensively in skin diseases generally and is thought by many to be superior to sarsaparilla.

It is an excellent blood purifier and it will clear up all kinds of skin symptoms, but it must be continued for a long period. It is excellent for boils and abscesses. For

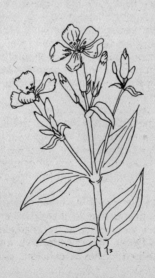

much irritation of the skin a strong decoction of the root may be applied as often as is necessary.

Directions for use: 1 pint of boiling water should be poured on to 2 ozs. of the dried leaves or root; when cold this should be strained and 1 or 2 tablespoonsful should be taken three or four times daily.

A strong decoction is made by boiling 2 ozs. of the powdered root in 1 pint of water down to half a pint of liquid which should then be strained.

TANSY
(Tanacetum vulgare)

Also known as Buttons.

Description: This herb is found growing in hedgerows and on waste ground; it has oblong leaves which grow alternately up the stem which is about 2 to 3 ft tall; the leaves are about 4 inches wide, deeply divided like a feather, dark green with about twelve pointed serrated segments on either side. The stem branches at the top on which are flat topped bright yellow heads. The leaves smell like camphor.

Part used: The herb.

The name comes from *Athanasia*, an ancient word for immortality, because it flowers for a very long time.

The taste is aromatic and the shredded leaves were employed until a short time ago, and may still be in some country districts, for flavouring cakes and puddings.

Tansy cakes were made in olden days and eaten during Lent in remembrance of the bitter herbs taken at the Passover. They were served at the coronation feast of James II and his Queen Mary of Modena, together with some fifteen hundred 'dishes of delicious viands includ-

ing four fauns, stag's tongues, gotwits; brown buds and
taffeta tarts'.

'This Balsemic plant,' said Boerhaave, 'will supply the
place of nutmegs and cinnamon'.

Tansy is an old well-known family remedy used to
tone up the system.

It is good for some eruptive conditions of the skin and
hot fomentations wrung out of tansy tea are excellent
for inflammations, bruising, freckles and sunburn.

Tansy tea should be taken freely instead of the usual
Indian variety and it is excellent for the skin and many
blemishes.

Directions for use: To drink as a tea put 1½ teaspoonsful
in a 1½ pint teapot and infuse for five or six minutes
before drinking. The flavour is slightly tart and peppery.
An infusion is made by pouring 1 pint of boiling water
on to 1 oz. of the herb and a wineglassful taken freely.

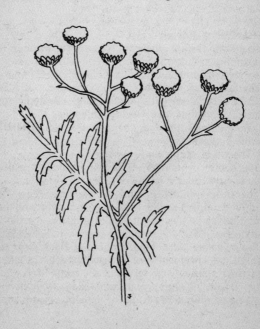

WALNUT
(Juglans nigra)

Description: The leaflets vary in size on the same leaf, which has seven to nine leaflets — they are from 2¼ to 4 inches in length and 1 to 1½ inches wide, parchment like when dry, leafstalks brown. The bark occurs in curved pieces 3 to 6 inches long and about 1 inch broad, dull, blackish brown, tough, fibrous and mealy. The taste of both leaves and bark is bitter but the odour of the leaves is aromatic.

Part used: The bark and leaves.

It is not known exactly when walnut trees were brought to Britain but Pepys wrote: 'To Nonsuch, to the Exchequer by appointment, and walked up and down the house and park . . . a great walk of an elme and a walnutt set one after another in that order . . . ' Nonsuch was one of Henry's VIII's great palaces which indicates the trees were probably planted in his reign.

Walnut trees live to a great age and it is said that there is one in Balaclava around one thousand years old.

The roots, leaves and rind yield a brown dye which is supposed to contain iodine and which gipsies employ for staining their skins. It also dyes the hair black.

Culpeper said: 'The kernels, when they grow old, are more oily and unfit to be eaten, but are then used to heal the wounds of the sinews, gangrenes and carbuncles'. And, 'The distilled water of the green leaves in the end of May, cures foul running ulcers and sores to be bathed with wet cloths or sponges applied to them every morning'.

Dr. Fernie said: 'The walnut has been justly termed vegetable arsenic because of it's curative virtues in eczema and other obstinate conditions of the skin'.

This is excellent in the treatment of herpes and when there is burning and itching of the skin of an eczematous nature lasting a long time and leaving the affected parts blue and swollen.

Directions for use: An infusion is made by pouring 1 pint of boiling water on 1 oz. of the bark or leaves. This mixture should be strained when cool and a wineglassful taken three times daily. This same infusion may be applied externally to all skin eruptions.

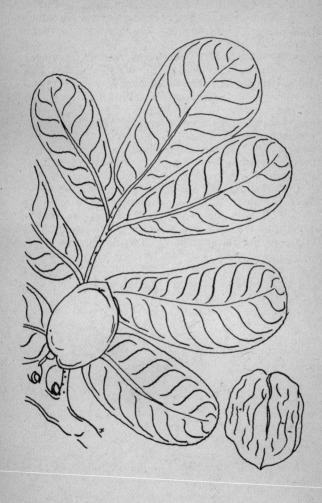

WILD STRAWBERRY
(Fragaria vesca)

Also known as Mountain strawberry, Woodberry, Pine-apple strawberry.

Description: This is a familiar little plant with trifoliate leaves and white flowers with scarlet or crimson fruits.

Part used: The leaves.

The word strawberry is from the anglo-saxon *Streow-berie* of which the first syllable refers to anything strewn. Another source says the plant gets its familiar name from the straw which is placed between the rows to protect the fruit from being splashed by the soil.

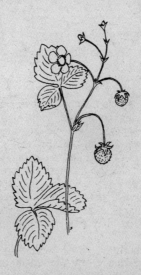

The wild woodland strawberry is the progenitor of our highly cultivated and delicious fruit.

Thomas Tusser wrote:
'If frost do continue, take this for a law,
The strawberries look to be covered with straw!'

Gerard said: 'The leaves boiled and applied in manner of a pultis taketh away the burning heate in wounds . . . the ripe strawberries quench thirst and take away if they be often used, the rednesse and heate of the face'.

This herb is good for eczema and should be applied externally as well as taken internally.

Directions for use: Add 1 oz. of the leaves to 1 pint of boiling water and infuse for ten minutes. A wineglassful should be taken three times daily.

This should also be applied to the skin externally.

WILD THYME
(Thymus serpyllum)

Also known as Brotherwort, Creeping thyme, Mother thyme.

Description: It grows on hills, heaths and in meadows and is a creeping evergreen. This plant has a small stringy, creeping root, from which rise a great number of very slender, woody stalks, having two small, roundish, green leaves, set at a joint on short footstalks. The flowers grow on the top of the stalks among the leaves, in small loose spikes of a reddish purple colour. The leaves and flowers have a very sweet scent. The appearance of this herb varies slightly in different soils — some leaves may be dark green and others more hairy.

Part used: The herb.

Thyme is derived from the greek word *thumos* —

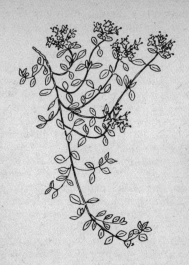

meaning smoke — as it was used in sacrifices because of its fragrant odour. The Greeks name thyme as their emblem of bravery and activity.

Francis Bacon said that the plants 'which do perfume the air most delightfully, not passed by as the rest, but trodden upon and crushed are three, burnet, wild thyme and water mint'. He also wrote of his garden 'I like also little heaps, in the nature of mole-hills to be set, some with wild thyme, some with pinks and some with germander'.

The delicious flavour of the honey of Hymettus was said to be derived from the wild thyme there, visited by the bees.

This herb is an excellent tonic and an infusion is good if applied for the healing of various skin eruptions.

Directions for use: An infusion should be made with ½ oz. of the dried herb to which has been added ½ pint of boiling water and applied to the skin freely when cold.

It should be taken as a tea and made by pouring 1½ pints of boiling water on to a teaspoonful of the dried herb and allowed to stand for five minutes before drinking. It may be sweetened with a little honey if desired.

YELLOW DOCK
(Rumex crispus)

Also known as Sour dock, curled dock, garden patience.
Description: Grows freely in roadside ditches and on waste ground. The leaves are narrow and oblong, and crisped at the margins. Sepals hang down from short individual stalks from the main stem in groups of five or six. The root occurs in short shrivelled pieces ¾ to 1 inch long, brown, rough and wrinkled.
Part used: The root.

This plant is called the yellow curled dock because the leaves are crisped at the edges.

Culpeper said: 'The roots boiled in vinegar helpeth the itch, scabs and breaking out of the skin if it be bathed therewith. The distilled water of the herb and roots have the same virtue and cleanseth the skin from freckles, morphews and all other spots and discolourings therein'.

This herb is an excellent blood purifier; at the same time it tones up the system.

It helps eruptive diseases of the skin and is soothing for constant itching.

Dr. Fernie recommends an ointment made from the yellow dock and gives the following instructions for making it: 'an ointment may be made by boiling the root in vinegar until the fibre is softened and by then mixing this pulp with lard (to which some sulphur is added)'. This is excellent for itching and sores.

Also a strong infusion may be applied as often as is necessary for skin troubles with intense irritation.

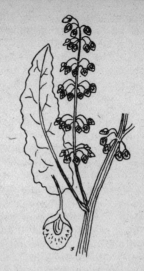

Directions for use: 1 pint of boiling water should be added to 1 oz. of the powdered root; when cold this should be strained and wineglassful doses taken three times daily.

For the strong infusion to be applied externally, pour 1 pint of boiling water on to a large handful of the freshly gathered leaves; pour off when cold and apply freely.

SUPPLEMENTARY ADVICE

There is no doubt that a good healthy and cleansing diet plays a part in the elimination of all skin troubles.

It cannot be emphasized too strongly that fresh fruit, salads and conservatively cooked fresh vegetables should be eaten every day. Eggs, cheese, chicken, lamb or a small steak should be taken in moderation to give protein. If potatoes are eaten they should be cooked in their jackets because the mineral salts are found just under the skin. To peel a potato robs it of its nutritive value.

Cottage cheese is very good and can be flavoured with herbs such as chives; cheddar cheese may be taken, but the very highly flavoured varieties should be avoided.

Fresh fruit should be taken at all times instead of pies and puddings. Salads should contain as many of the following as are obtainable: lettuce, watercress, mustard and cress, grated cabbage (the white variety is most suitable), shredded raw beetroot, raw onion rings or spring onions, cucumber, radishes, tomatoes, grated raw carrot. A desertspoonful of sunflower seed oil should be taken daily poured over the salad.

Only 100 per cent. wholemeal bread should be eaten, unless too much roughage cannot be tolerated for reasons of ulceration and other causes. Then bread made from an 81 per cent. extraction is the next best thing.

Foods that should be omitted from the diet of all sufferers from skin troubles are milk, buttermilk, yoghourt, cream, bananas, dried fruits, honey and any form of sweetening, also condiments and salty foods.

Butter should be taken sparingly.

Tea and coffee should be avoided and replaced by herbal teas, already discussed in this book. Hot Vecon or Marmite may be taken, or decaffinated or dandelion coffee.

Vitamin deficiency is sometimes responsible for eczema, psoriasis and boils, the body usually being short of A, the B complex and C.

It is wise, therefore, to take a course of these vitamins and it is suggested that one capsule of 100 mgms of vitamin C should be taken daily with any one meal.

Foods rich in vitamin C are: rose-hips, pimentos, turnip tops, brussel sprouts, dandelion leaves, grapefruit, oranges, tangerines, cabbage, black currants, straw-berries, kale, broccoli, parsley, watercress and tomatoes.

Vitamin A is also necessary and is richest in the following foods: halibut liver oil, cod liver oil, calves liver, dairy goods, dandelion leaves, carrots, endive, raw apricots, turnip tops, spinach, tomato puree, kale and parsley.

A course of halibut liver oil daily would be helpful.

Brewers yeast is the cheapest and easiest way to take the B vitamins. The best way for the beginner is to add no more than 1 teaspoonful to a large glass of fruit juice. This should be increased gradually to 2 or 3 teaspoonsful daily.

Essential fatty acids are also necessary for a healthy body and skin. This is why the sunflower seed oil is recommended to be taken with salads, otherwise 2 ounces of the seeds should be chewed well and eaten daily.

The average skin will not tolerate too many hot baths; in any case, these are enervating and should be avoided. Warm or tepid baths should be taken and then the skin rubbed briskly with a rough towel.

At the same time avoid all strong soaps and use instead one of the herbal soaps which are preferable.

Fresh air is most important, as is daily exercise, especially a good walk. Strong sunlight is not good for some skin eruptions and should be avoided.

Warm but light clothing is ideal in the winter, remember that the skin has to 'breathe' and the pores are inclined to get 'clogged' if smothered with too much heavy clothing.

And one final warning: do not cook any food, boil any liquids, or infuse any herbs in aluminium utensils as they can be detrimental to health.

THERAPEUTIC INDEX

Abscess, Brooklime, Scurvy grass, Soapwort.
Bites, Echinachea.
Blemishes, Garlic, Lady's mantle, Nettle, Tansy.
Blood Purifier, Bittersweet, Burdock, Chickweed, Clivers, Dandelion, Echinacea, Garlic, Nettle, Red clover, Sassafras, Soapwort, Yellow dock.
Blotches, Garlic.
Boils, Brooklime, Burdock, Chickweed, Echinacea, Plantain, Scurvy grass, Soapwort.
Bruising, Tansy.
Burns, Bilberry, Bittersweet, Brooklime, Burdock, Chickweed, Houseleek, Marshmallow, Nettle, Plantain.
Carbuncles, Burdock, Echinacea, Garlic, Plantain, Walnut.
Corns, Celandine, Houseleek.
Eczema, Burdock, Celandine, Clivers, Dandelion, Nettle, Plantain, Walnut, Wild strawberry.
Erysipelas, Houseleek, Plantain.
External Applications, Bilberry, Bittersweet, Brooklime, Celandine, Chickweed, Clivers, Houseleek, Lady's mantle, Marshmallow, Nettle, Plantain, Red clover, Soapwort, Tansy, Walnut, Wild strawberry, Wild thyme, Yellow dock.
Freckles, Fumitory, Tansy.
Herpes, Walnut.
Irritation, Soapwort.
Itching, Burdock, Celandine, Clivers, Dandelion, Nettle, Plantain, Walnut, Wild strawberry, Yellow dock.
Nettle Rash, Nettle.
Pimples, Brooklime, Fumitory, Garlic, Scurvy grass.

Scabs, Chickweed, Fumitory, Marshmallow, Plantain, Scurvy grass, Yellow dock.

Scalds, Bilberry, Bittersweet, Chickweed, Houseleek, Marshmallow, Plantain.

Shingles, Houseleek, Plantain.

Sores, Chickweed, Echinacea, Lady's mantle, Marshmallow, Plantain, Red clover, Scurvy grass, Walnut, Yellow dock.

Stings, Echinacea, Houseleek, Marshmallow, Plantain.

Styes, Burdock.

Sunburn, Tansy.

Tonic, Buckbean, Wild thyme.

Ulcers, Brooklime, Plantain, Walnut.

Warts, Celandine.

Whitlows, Brooklime.

Wounds, Burdock, Chickweed, Echinacea, Lady's mantle, Red clover, Shepherd's purse.